I0693788

PREGNANCY DIET MAGIC

Delicious and Nutritious Recipes to Nourish Your Growing Baby

Kristie Fleming

This book Belongs to

____

Baby's name

____

TABLE OF CONTENTS

INTRODUCTION

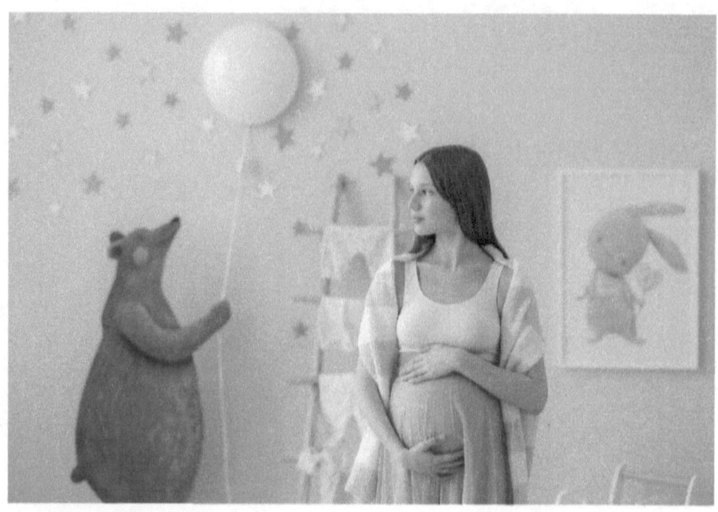

There are numerous fantasies encompassing the eating routine for pregnant moms. We frequently hear the older folks of the family encouraging youthful moms

to eat enough for two people. Today, we realize that this isn't accurate. As a matter of fact, unrestrained eating during pregnancy can make you put on a great deal of weight and can make your kid superfluously overweight. What then could be the best eating regimen for pregnant ladies?

The developing hatchling gets generally Its

sustenance from its mom through the umbilical rope. Consequently, while the mother doesn't need to eat sufficient nourishment for two people, she actually should accept in an adequate number of supplements for two people. Assuming the mother experiences supplement lack, this will be given to the youngster. Early supplement lack can prompt various formative issues in small kids.

The pregnancy diet should be wealthy in every one of the fundamental supplements that the body needs. Specialists prescribe the admission of six to seven servings of bread and grains, two to four servings of natural product, four to six servings of vegetables, two to four servings of dairy and roughly three servings of protein consistently. It is generally fitting to pick food that is wealthy in fiber. Fantastic models incorporate entire grain oats, rice, products of the soil green veggies.

Calcium is essential to the development of bones and teeth. Make sure to take in something like four servings of calcium rich dairy items. This will guarantee that you *get roughly 1200 mg of calcium consistently. The eating regimen of pregnant ladies ought to be wealthy in iron.*

L-ascorbic acid reinforces the insusceptible arrangement of the mother and kid. Significant wellsprings of L-ascorbic acid incorporate citrus natural products, broccoli, cauliflower, papaya, green peppers and tomatoes.

Vitamin An is similarly significant. Carrots, yams, spinach, turnip, apricots and water squash contain loads of vitamin A.

An eager mother should constantly accept all her endorsed pre-birth nutrients. These are exceptionally concocted multivitamins that make up for any supplement lopsided characteristics or lacks in the mother's eating regimen. By and large, these contain iron, minerals, nutrients, folic corrosive and calcium. The lack of folic corrosive can prompt serious birth imperfection in children. Green verdant vegetables, nuts, citrus leafy foods are plentiful in regular folic corrosive, nutrients and iron.

Similarly as there are things that should be remembered for the eating regimen for *pregnant ladies, there are sure things that should be stayed away from during pregnancy. These incorporate liquor, caffeine, excess sugar, excess fat and crude meat. It is prudent to keep away from delicate cheddar, and to swear off eating shark, swordfish and mackerel which elevated degrees of mercury in them.*

Most pregnant moms feel queasiness and a discouraging absence of hunger during their most memorable trimester. At this stage, they might eat little feasts over the course of the day.

Numerous ladies put on a great deal of weight because of the great fat, salt and sugar content in their pregnancy diet. It is actually the case that pregnant ladies frequently go areas of strength for through and sharp cravings for food. In any case, assuming you want to monitor your weight and shed additional pounds rapidly after conveyance, then, at that point, it is vital to eat food sources low in calories and high in nutritive worth.

Eating Right During Pregnancy

Pregnancy is a multi month venture… It is a period in your life to feel blissful, energized, peaceful and happy. Anyway it is additionally very common to encounter tensions about the birth and agonizing over whether you are feeding yourself appropriately, working out, keeping, quiet, positive, cherishing contemplations and feelings inside your being.

Pregnancy endures 39 weeks or nine months from origination and is checked in three phases out.

CHAPTER 1: EATING WELL DURING PREGNANCY

To guarantee that your child creates in a sound climate, you ought to keep your body as fit and very much fed as you can. Try not to think as far as contriving an exceptional eating regimen for pregnancy, it is more to do with eating a decent assortment of the right food varieties which are those that are wealthy in the fundamental supplements.

Weight Gain

How much weight put on by ladies in pregnancy

fluctuates between 9 - 16 kilograms, with the most fast addition typically between weeks 24 and 32.

Try not to "eat for two". Around 46% of ladies gain an excess of weight during pregnancy.

Diet During Pregnancy

The type of food you eat will affect you general health in this manner Your Child Is What You Eat!

What You Eat influences your child's future. What you eat in the accompanying nine months can affect your child's wellbeing, as well as your own, long into the future.

A decent eating routine Is crucial to wellbeing during pregnancy, and to the ordinary improvement of the child. An opportunity to focus on diet, and if essential improve it, is a while preceding origination and not when pregnancy is affirmed.

During the basic early weeks the typical, solid advancement of the undeveloped organism relies upon the mother's condition of nourishing wellbeing and furthermore her harmful state.

Mineral and nutrient uneven characters which would likely slip through the cracks in a youngster or grown-up can lamentably affect the creating child.

This is on the grounds that the cells in the undeveloped organism are developing at a particularly fast rate, making a misrepresented reaction any destructive impacts.

A characteristic, natural, entire food diet is the one in particular which will enough serve during pregnancy.

A top notch diet is expected to keep up with your own wellbeing and the most ideal circumstances for the child to create.

As our current circumstance turns out to be more contaminated and the dirts more drained of supplements, going 100 percent natural, on the off chance that conceivable, is the most ideal option for oneself, and for a creating hatchling, and to wrap things up; the climate.

Pesticides, herbicides, and different types of contamination disrupt the metabolic pathways of numerous supplements and in this way in a roundabout way obstruct the improvement of the resistant, endocrine, and neurological frameworks.

Eating as a significant number of our food sources in their live, crude structure jam 70 to 80% more nutrients and minerals, half more bioactive protein, and up to 96% more bioavailable vitamin B12.

Grains, nuts and seeds are the most intense wellbeing building food sources of all. Eaten crude or grew if conceivable (a few grains should be cooked), they contain every one of the fundamental supplements for human development, food, and continuous ideal wellbeing.

An even eating regimen depends on entire cereals and grains (earthy colored *bread, rice, pasta, buckwheat, rye, oats), nuts and seeds, heartbeats and beans, new leafy foods, unadulterated raw oils like virus squeezed olive oil, with some fish and eggs whenever required.*

Products of the soil are astounding wellsprings of nutrients, minerals and minor components gave they are eaten in the correct manner.

It would be ideal for they to be new, either crude or immediately cooked, steamed or sautéed, and ideally consumed following they are reaped.

Salt is expected to keep up with the additional volume of blood, to supply sufficient placental blood, and to prepare for parchedness and shock from blood misfortune upon entering the world, (besides in instances of kidney and heart issues) Recommended type of salt is Himalayan Pink Salt.

Proteins

ï¿½ Structure the essential structure blocks of all our body tissues, cells, chemicals, and antibodies.

ï¿½ Food should fuel the development of the uterus,

which can develop to multiple times its unique size over the nine months growth period Add the improvement of bosoms, placenta, advancement of bosom milk, the child's body.

Proteins are separated into complete and deficient:

Complete proteins contain huge measures of the multitude of fundamental *amino acids, you find them in meat, poultry, fish, eggs, milk and soya bean items.*

Vegetable proteins are fragmented and contain just a portion of the fundamental amino acids. Some vegan wellsprings of complete protein are: buckwheat, sesame seeds, pumpkin seeds, sunflower seeds, flaxseeds, and almonds.

Plant proteins are simpler for our bodies to process and create less harmful material than creature proteins. The fiber in plants likewise affects the gut; it guarantees solid defecations and the right bacterial populace in the stomach, and forestalls the development of putrefactive microbes delivered by abundance creature proteins.

Eating meat and meat items additionally conveys the gamble from substance and hormonal deposits tracked down in seriously raised creatures. Additionally soya beans or soy items are for the most part hereditarily designed, subsequently avoiding them is savvy.

Pregnant ladies need around 60 to 75 grams of protein daily.

The best and cleanest wellsprings of protein are green vegetables, spirulina, seeds (hemp, flax, sesame, poppy, sunflower, chia, quinoa, amaranth).

Genuine strength and building material comes from:

ï¿½ green - verdant vegetables, seeds and superfoods. They contain every one of the amino acids we require.

Fundamental Unsaturated fats are imperative to:

ï¿½ the improvement of the child's apprehensive and resistant frameworks. They assemble the cell walls in the entirety of our tissues, thus that minor components and fat-dissolvable nutrients (A,E,D, and K) can be assimilated.

ï¿½ EFA's are expected to make adrenal and sex chemicals, and to keep a solid populace of microscopic organisms in the stomach.

ï¿½ They are additionally vital for the typical advancement of the baby's mind: 70% of all EFAs go to the cerebrum.

The Best Greasy Food varieties include:

Avocados, Borage Seed Oil, Crude Cacao Beans (Chocolate Nuts), Coconut oil/spread, Flax seed and its oil, Grape seeds, Hemp seed and its oil (cold squeezed), Crude Nuts of numerous types (cashews should be delicate to develop be really "crude"), Nut Margarines (almond spread is superb), Olives and their oil (stone squeezed or cold squeezed), Peanuts (should be ensured aflatoxin free), Poppy seeds, pumpkin seeds and their oil (cold squeezed), Sesame seeds, sunflower seeds, tahini (sesame margarine), or far superior in the event that you can get hold of it at a wellbeing food store unhulled tahini (a soluble fat, high in calcium), Youthful Coconuts (youthful

Thai coconuts are accessible in the US at Asian business sectors), Coconut milk, coconuts).

SUPERFOODS

Superfoods are food sources with unprecedented properties. Normally they contain all fundamental amino acids, elevated degrees of minerals, and a wide exhibit of one of a kind, even intriguing, supplements. I have incorporated the superfoods in the healthful tips underneath.

Some unmistakable superfoods to include:

1) Himalayan Pink Salt - offers 84 minerals precisely indistinguishable from the components in your body.

2)   *Spirulina (a twisting green growth consumed for millennia by native individuals in Mexico and Africa)*

-It has the most noteworthy grouping of protein on The planet. 60%

-It is additionally extremely high in Iron, and numerous different nutrients and minerals.

-It is one of the greatest wellsprings of gamma-linolenic corrosive (GLA) in the world. Just mother's milk is higher.

-It is prescribed to take more Spirulina during breastfeeding on account of the GLA.

-Spirulina is exceptionally high in human-dynamic B12.

3)   *Blue Green growth (Klamath lake green growth great cerebrum food). It is high in protein, chlorophyll, nutrients, and minerals and improves the safe framework.*

I esteem it in pre-pregnancy, pregnancy, and lactation for its upgrading impact on mind capability.

4)   Bee Dust (wild dust, not plantation dust, ought to be utilized and ought to come from morally reaped sources where honey bees are dealt with deferentially. Honey bee Dust is nature's most finished food) Every amino corrosive, resistant framework, cerebrum, eyes.

5)   Flax, Sunflower, Chia, Sesame and pumpkin seeds are awesome to utilize. Flaxseeds are

fantastic and the most noteworthy vegan wellspring of omega-3-fundamental unsaturated fats, significant for the invulnerable framework, sensory system, and mental health. I prescribe one to two tablespoons everyday of the uncooked and unheated oil or three to six tablespoons of newly ground flaxseeds. (Utilize an espresso processor). You may likewise crush the other previously mentioned seeds and add them to plates of mixed greens, and organic product servings of mixed greens.

6) Wild youthful coconuts (not be mistaken for white Thai coconuts found in business sectors, wild coconuts are quite possibly of the best food on the planet. The coconut water and delicate internal tissue

are strength improving, electrolyte-rich, mineral-rich, youthening and animating. Extraordinary in smoothies.

Sustenance TIPS

Here Are Some Sustenance Tips that will help you both:

1)   Get Enough Folic Corrosive. 400 micrograms (mcg) everyday. Folic Corrosive diminishes

chance of birth deformities, for example, spina bifida. Particularly in the initial a month and a half of pregnancy.

2)   Best Food Wellsprings of Folic Corrosive are: Crude Green verdant vegetables, including spinach, kale, beet greens, beet root, chard, asparagus, and broccoli. Boring vegetables containing folic corrosive are corn, lima

beans, green peas, sweet peas, yams, artichokes, okra, and parsnips. Oats are high in folic corrosive as well as entire wheat earthy colored bread. Many natural products have folic corrosive like oranges, melon, pineapple, banana, and many berries including loganberries, boysenberries, and strawberries. Likewise new fledglings, for example, lentil, mung bean sprouts are phenomenal sources. *Update: Folic corrosive is accessible from new, natural food, which is the reason it is so normal a lacking in our way of life's handled, prepared food diet.*

3)   Eat Your Fish. *Getting enough DHA (tracked down in overflow in fish and flaxseed) is perhaps of the main thing you can accomplish for yourself as well as your fostering child's*

wellbeing. DHA is the omega-3 unsaturated fat that can help child's mental health before birth, prompting better vision, memory, coordinated movements and language appreciation in youth. Eat no less than 12 ounces every seven day stretch of low-mercury fish, or take a DHA supplement, for example, Krill Oil.

ï¿½ Stay away from huge, savage fish like shark, swordfish, lord mackerel and tilefish. (As hotshot eat more modest fish, the bigger, longer-living ones collect more mercury).

ï¿½ Kelp and Cilantro eliminate weighty metals and radioactive isotopes from the tissues.

4) Avoid Liquor - The primary gamble of drinking

liquor during pregnancy is the improvement of "fetal liquor condition" (FAS). Mother.. NO Sum IS Protected. Keep away from Completely.

5)   Avoid Caffeine: In high sums causes birth imperfections yet births, unsuccessful labors and unexpected labor.

6)   Avoid Medications - Quite far all customary

medications ought to be kept away from during pregnancy, particularly in the initial three months. Think about normal other options and visiting a clinical cultivator or nutritionist before origination.

Food varieties THAT Might CAUSE Diseases

Albeit the possibility contracting one of these

uncommon diseases is restricted, you will lessen this probability considerably further in the event that you keep the essential rules given here.

Listeriosis - brought about by the bacterium Listeria monocytogenes, this is an exceptionally interesting contamination. Its side effects are like influenza and gastroenteritis and it can cause actually birth.

Toxoplasmosis - typically symptomless (aside from gentle influenza side effects), this can lead to difficult issues for the child. Brought about by direct contact with the living being Toxoplasma Gondi, it is tracked down in feline defecation, crude meat, and unpasteurized goats' milk. Soil on leafy foods might be polluted.

Salmonella - Tainting with Salmonella bacterium can cause bacterial food contamination. This doesn't as a rule hurt the child straightforwardly, however any disease including a high temperature, heaving, looseness of the bowels, and parchedness could cause an unnatural birth cycle or preterm work.

Natural cures are generally very protected to be taken during pregnancy; some are helpful options in contrast to drugs both in ongoing disease and intense minor issues, for example, may emerge during pregnancy. It is as yet desirable over take NO Drug at all in the initial three months, except if there is a particular issue that needs treatment.

There are numerous Spices which ought to never be taken in pregnancy - their emmonagogue or oxytocic properties may, in huge sums, cause uterine constrictions and subsequently risk premature delivery: I will just specify a couple as there something like twenty on the rundown.

Nutmeg Myristica Fragrans

Thuja occidentalis

Calendula officinalis

Sage Salvia officinalis

Thyme Thymus vulgaris

Marjoram Origanum vulgare

Lovage Levisticum officinale

Rosemary Rosmarinus Officinalis

Rhubarb Rheum sp.

Spices that are protected to eat to take in culinary portions however not as a medication during pregnancy include:

Celery seed, cinnamon, fennel, fenugreek, oregano, parsley, rosemary, sage and saffron.

CHAPTER 2: HEALTHY FOODS TO EAT DURING PREGNANCY

Each mother needs to have a simple, straightforward pregnancy and a sound kid. Tragically, an ever increasing number of ladies experience pregnancy inconveniences, for example, weakness, hypertension, thyroid issues, diabetes, unexpected labor, and low birth weight.

More youngsters are brought into the world with birth abandons and a significant number of the people who seem ordinary upon entering the world proceed to foster medical conditions further down the road.

One of every 10 children will have ADHD, one out of 150 will become medically introverted. Kids are impacted by tension, sorrow, and bipolar problem. Kids foster sort 2 diabetes, which was incomprehensible only a long time back.

Specialists concur that the greater part of these issues can be decreased and, surprisingly, forestalled by *legitimate sustenance during pregnancy.*

Mother's sustenance has an influence not just on the pregnancy and on the baby's introduction to the world weight, yet even on the gamble of birth surrenders, pregnancy complexities, maternal ailment, and future infections when the youngster turns into a grown-up.

Supplements diminish pregnancy difficulties and birth surrenders

Concentrates on show that legitimate eating regimen and dietary enhancements, for example, fish oil, nutrients C and E can forestall mother's ailment during pregnancy and untimely birth. Vitamin An and beta-carotene alongside magnesium, fish oil, and zinc can lessen maternal mortality. Iron and folic corrosive lessen paleness. Calcium lessens the rate of toxemia and hypertension.

As indicated by the Diary of Nourishment:

"Various examinations support the idea that a significant reason for pregnancy inconveniences can be poor nourishment."

"Recurrence and seriousness of pregnancy confusions might be diminished through an improvement in the supplement status of the mother."

"Maternal healthful lacks … might be huge supporters of the event of birth absconds."

Maternal sustenance will influence the remainder of the youngster's life

Clinical examination demonstrates the way that great sustenance during pregnancy and youth can lessen child's gamble of future malignant growth.

Legitimate maternal nourishing supplementation can decrease the endanger of diabetes later in youngster's life.

Certain particular inadequacies (for instance magnesium) can likewise build the gamble of future diabetes.

Indeed, even the gamble of future osteoporosis (in a child when the person turns into a grown) not entirely settled by "maternal healthful status during pregnancy" and particularly by lack of vitamin D, which is exceptionally normal.

Most pregnant ladies are insufficient

Tragically, most pregnant ladies are lacking in nutrients, minerals, amino acids, and omega 3 unsaturated fats.

Omega 3 unsaturated fats, particularly DHA, are

essential for the cerebrum, focal sensory system, and the retina. A child needs them for ordinary improvement of the cerebrum and the eyes.

Untimely newborn children are bound to have ADHD, wretchedness, and schizophrenia, on the grounds that their minds didn't get an opportunity to completely create and integrate all the DHA it required. Then again, offspring of moms who eat enormous measure of greasy fish have better savvy advancement and higher intelligence levels.

The issue is that practically 90% of ladies don't get even the insignificant measure of DHA. Numerous ladies are lacking in folic corrosive, in spite of food fortress. Lacks of magnesium, calcium, iron, vitaminsC, D, E, and numerous different supplements are exceptionally normal, which can imperil the soundness of both the mother and the child.

Try not to rely on pre-birth multivitamin - it doesn't work

The miserable truth is that a regular remedy pre-birth lacks of nutrient doesn't *right most, which are common to pregnant women*

Pre-birth multivitamin is an unfortunate wellspring of supplements. Every one of the fixings are manufactured, so your body can't utilize them the manner in which it utilizes regular supplements from food.

Additionally it is stacked with synthetic substances, for example, crospovidone, FD&C Red No. 40 aluminum lake, hydroxypropyl methylcellulose, lactose, magnesium stearate, mineral oil light, polysorbate 80, sodium lauryl sulfate, stearic corrosive, syloid, titanium dioxide and triethyl citrate. Neither you nor your child need these synthetic compounds. They don't help, however can hurt.

How might you make certain to have the most ideal sustenance

Eat a decent eating regimen. This implies eat normal food varieties. Oats is normal, yet grain produced using oats that appears as though little doughnuts isn't. Steak is regular, however lunch meeting meat isn't. Eggs are regular, eggbeaters are manufactured unnatural garbage.

As such, eat food how it is normally delivered and stay away from handled, man-made food varieties. This typically implies keeping away from anything that comes in boxes, jars, and plastic bundles and whatever has lapse date a long time from today.

Genuine food ruins, low quality food is stacked with additives, so it can keep going for quite a while.

Eat products of the soil, nuts and seeds, berries, meat, chicken, sheep, eggs, cheddar, spread, and whatever other regular food that you like. Fish and fish are normally alright, however eat enormous fish (salmon, fish, and so on) with some restraint in view of possibly high mercury content.

Attempt to limit pop, frozen yogurt, treats, white bread and white rice, most breakfast cereals, and some other handled food varieties.

However, in any event, eating a decent eating regimen might be leave you lacking in significant supplements. For that reason I suggest nourishing enhancements.

As I referenced, pre-birth nutrients that you specialist recommended is only garbage. It is a blend of engineered synthetic substances, some of which might try and be unsafe for the creating child.

You ought to take just enhancements that are produced using genuine *food. There is an organization called Standard Interaction that has been delivering food-based supplements since 1920s. They develop foods grown from the ground on their own ensured natural homestead. They get dried out them utilizing a licensed low-heat high-vacuum process that holds every one of the supplements. Consider it transforming a grape into a raisin. Raisins have generally similar supplements as grapes, with the exception of water.*

They likewise use organ meats (liver, kidney, and so forth) from natural cows since they have exceptionally high supplement content. They join various fixings to make different nourishing enhancements. There isn't anything fake, no additives, no synthetics, just genuine food with genuine supplements.

It Is never too soon or past the time to begin. Whether you are simply arranging your pregnancy or are in the third trimester, you want legitimate nourishment at each stage.

This is the program I prescribe to my patients:

· *Catalyn - a characteristic multivitamin/multimineral produced using 12 unique food sources*

· *Folic Corrosive B12 - for extra folic corrosive and B12*

· *Ferrofood - regular natural iron*

· *Calcium lactate - regular calcium and magnesium from beats*

· *TunaOmega oil - normally unadulterated wellspring of DHA and EPA, ensured liberated from mercury, PCBs, and different synthetic compounds*

CHAPTER 3: FOODS TO AVOID DURING PREGNANCY

No time is sustenance more significant in a lady's life than when she is having a child. This time is laden with stresses over getting an adequate number of nutrients and minerals and not eating anything destructive.

The more we are asking to be aware of our food sources and what synthetics are going in them *and on them the more unfortunate we become as moms. Trans fats, soaked fats, unpasteurized milks, reconstituted corn syrup, hereditarily changed soy bean, mercury in fish, pesticides on natural products, sugar, salts; it is essentially unimaginable o comprehend what a mother ought to eat.*

The following is a rundown of simple to keep guidelines

for keeping away from unsafe eating during pregnancy:

1.   Avoid reconstituted anything: read the names assuming you see reconstitutes corn syrup, natural product squeeze, any fixing set the item back on the rack. Reconstituted implies they took the crude fixings transformed them here and there and utilized what was passed on to make this item. It is hard to express out loud whatever nature of fixings is being utilized when something has been reconstituted. During your pregnancy it is a lot more secure to go for item utilizing entire fixings like new organic product juices without added substances.

2.   Calcium is so significant in pregnancy. You really want around 1,500 mg of calcium consistently to supply enough to the hatchling for bone development and forestalls losing bone thickness. The best wellspring of calcium is most certainly dairy for however long it is sanitized. Cheeses, creams, milks, yogurt, frozen yogurt can be in every way eaten with some restraint assuming you check the name and it plainly expresses the item has been sanitized.

Assuming you are uncertain attempt tofu, salmon or green verdant vegetables.

3.   Many ladies decide to avoid meats during their pregnancy. This isn't required. However, there are a couple of basic standards for protecting meats. Cook all meats completely, eat no meat crude or intriguing. Devoted store and handled meats, they can be a wellspring of listeriosis. Keep away from pre-stuffed meat things.

4.   Seafood can cause a few ladies caution yet, similar to meat, in the event that it is cooked appropriately it is protected. Stay away from any crude or half-cooked fish, like sushi. Keep away from neighborhood fish found during contamination admonitions. Canned fish is fine. Huge fish like swordfish and shark can contain mercury so picking an alternate kind during pregnancy might be ideal.

5.   Drink 2-3 liters of water a day. Most towns in created nations have totally safe drinking water yet to be protected you might need to get your water tried or put resources into a water channel. Keeping a container of chilled water in the edge can assist with

empowering a few ladies to drink all the more yet put resources into a glass bottle or an impeccable take jug to stay away from pollution from rehashed utilization of plastic containers.

6.   Go natural: the expense of natural food varieties can be restrictive for certain individuals and there is exceptionally restricted proof to show eating hereditarily adjusted food

varieties when pregnancy can influence your child yet there are likewise extremely restricted long haul concentrates on which demonstrate there are no drawn out influences from eating hereditarily altered food varieties while pregnant. In the event that there was each an opportunity to go natural it is during your pregnancy.

CHAPTER 4: NUTRITIONAL REQUIREMENTS DURING PREGNANCY

Most ladies ordinarily mull over utilizing food supplements when they are anticipating a kid. Ladies truly need to take every one of the essential safeguards prior to taking any drug during this vital piece of their lives.

GNLD Worldwide (Brilliant Neo-Life Diamite) is a worldwide association conveying natural wholefood sustenance enhancements to wellbeing cognizant people starting around 1958 and GNLD nourishing items are enthusiastically suggested for use by pregnant ladies and the individuals who are at present breastfeeding.

Support for all Ladies

GNLD offers an entire line of premium quality enhancements to offer supplement help for expecting ladies along with mothers who are nursing. These nutritionals can assist mothers with enhancing the key supplements that are important by mother and youngster. Pregnant ladies need a great deal of nourishing help, even subsequent to conceiving an offspring. Moms ought to recharge their inventory of supplements for the wellbeing of their little one.

Expert Imperativeness Pack

The GNLD Expert Imperativeness Pack is one

of a few multi-dietary items from GNLD. Each pack contains exactly the same healthy supplements you can get from a frequently suggested portion of new products of the soil, basically coming from the carotenoid complex substance. A reliable adjusted products of the soil diet further develops mother's blood flow and diminishes the possibilities of birth surrenders. Each pack contains a carotenoid intricate, one Tre en, and one Salmon Oil In addition to. As such; Expert Essentialness pack contains principal supplements that advances ideal pre-birth improvement.

Zinc (Chelated)

Each parent doesn't maintain that their babies should foster any birth surrenders, which makes zinc a significant mineral in mother's eating routine. This GNLD mineral item additionally incorporates chelated amino acids to make it simpler to retain. Besides the fact that it forestalls birth surrenders in babies, zinc likewise works on the general safe strength of a kid. Making it a significant component.

GNLD Recipe IV In addition to

One more recommended nourishing pack from the line of GNLD items is Equation IV In addition to. This suggested item offers every one of the fundamental nutrients, minerals, and folic corrosive that mums (and every other person) need. Mothers who need that additional explosion of energy to pummel pressure can get it from this nutrient power pack.

Cal-Mag + Vitamin D (Chelated)

This is one of the GNLD items that is frequently suggested for pregnant mums. Ladies need sound bones and teeth since they are more helpless to osteoporosis than men. This urgent nutrient and mineral enhancement *supplies the fundamental measures of both calcium and magnesium. Note that adequate measures of magnesium assists with uterine compression torment during when ladies are going to conceive an offspring.*

GNLD Nourishake Protein -

Moms need to have the legitimate measure of protein in their eating regimen. It basically assists in the creation of muscles, ligaments, chemicals, tendons, hair, cerebrum with tissuing, and nerves. It likewise supports one's energy. Nourishake Protein Savor comes three sweet flavors.

Precautionary measures

Despite the fact that these items are food based and safe, we prompt for pregnant mums to look for clinical guidance from their PCP prior to taking nutrient enhancements. This is particularly valid for the people who intend to take food supplements while on endorsed prescriptions.

Other GNLD items praised for pregnant moms incorporate L-ascorbic acid (Edge controlled), Vitamin E Complicated, Female Home grown Complex, and Garlic Allium Complex.

CHAPTER 5: EATING FOR YOUR BABY'S HEALTH

Eating great during pregnancy is significant in light of the fact that it influences the wellbeing of the mother and the youngster. The child needs a satisfactory stockpile of supplements to appropriately create. Not just this, an eager lady's body needs energy to adapt to the pregnancy side effects. In this manner, the dinners ought to comprise of different food varieties stacked with proteins as well as food sources containing starch.

1.   Adopt a Decent Eating regimen

With a couple of exemptions, you can keep on eating ordinary during pregnancy. Your eating regimen ought to incorporate vegetables, organic products, entire grains, dairy items and lean meats in a reasonable extent. Ladies are stressed over acquiring pounds during pregnancy.

Subsequently, they don't eat fats. One can eat fats in a restricted sum. Obstruction is a typical issue in pregnancy. Expanding the admission of fiber can free the issue from clogging.

2.   Eat Regular Feasts and Treats

A smart dieting plan ought to comprise of regular dinners and treats. It very well may be a small bunch of nuts, a cut of natural product or a glass of newly made juice. In the previous stages, ladies endure morning ailment and as they enter the third trimester, they are endure sharpness and acid reflux. The best arrangement is to eat little, continuous dinners. More modest dinners are simpler to process and can be perfect for ladies enduring morning ailment and causticity. It guarantees that the stomach remains full. It likewise keeps a tab on the quantity of calories you consume assisting you with keeping up with solid weight. Different snacks you can eat are humus with breads, low-fat yogurt, mixed greens, raisins, ham and kid carrots.

3.   Avoid Certain Food sources

Your body is more powerless against food-borne sicknesses during pregnancy. Devouring incorrectly food sources can cause serious medical conditions from acid reflux to premature delivery. It is fitting for pregnant females to keep away from sushi, crude eggs, Tilefish and swordfish. Surrender tobacco, liquor and espresso. Attempt to stay away from delicate cheddar except if it is made of unpasteurized milk. Skirt the franks and store meats for some time.

4.   Get more Iron and Folic Corrosive

Iron and folic corrosive are among the most fundamental supplements while conveying. Specialists for the most part endorse nutrient enhancements to *compensate for lacks of nutrient, yet it is dependably a superior choice to get supplements and nutrients in their regular structure. Dietary iron forestalls frailty in pregnant ladies. Salad greens, lean meats, peaches, kidney beans, raisins and apples are great dietary wellsprings of iron.*

All things considered, it forestalls birth absconds in the creating hatchling. Food sources wealthy in Folate incorporate mustard greens, avocado, oranges, strawberries, kidney beans, dark looked at peas, collard greens, spinach and broccoli. A great deal of grains are sustained with folic corrosive and safe for utilization during pregnancy.

5.   Drink a lot of water

As well as eating a solid and adjusted diet, you

ought to drink a lot of water. Liquids assist with flushing out poisons. Also, it forestalls lack of hydration. It keeps the skin looking new and graceful and keeps issues like dry skin under control.

The food you eat is your child's primary wellspring of nourishment. In this way, focus on all that you put into your mouth.

CHAPTER 6: UNDERSTANDING FOOD LABELS

Item name and portrayal
All food sources should have a precise name. For instance, a food called 'Strawberry Lunch room' should contain strawberries, not simply strawberry seasoning.

'Use by' or 'best before' date

Food varieties with a short life should have a 'utilization by' date. These food varieties are protected to eat until that date. Notwithstanding, this additionally relies upon right capacity. Capacity directions can likewise be tracked down on the name.

A food past Its 'utilization by' date ought not be sold.

It probably won't be protected to eat.

'Best before' signifies the food ought to keep up with its quality until that date. It could in any case be protected to eat after that time. Nonetheless, it could not. The food could have lost a portion of its flavor or sustenance.

A 'prepared on' or 'heated for' date is allowed for

bread. This is assuming its timeframe of realistic usability is under 7 days.

Food varieties that last north of 2 years, like canned food varieties, needn't bother with any date stamping.

Headings for capacity There can be directions for putting away food until its best-previously or use-by date. Any capacity conditions should be remembered for the name, for example,

Temperature
Dampness level
Conditions once the food is opened
Focusing on the capacity guidelines and practice great food arrangement hygiene is significant.

Fixings list

All fixings ought to be recorded arranged by weight in the food. The fundamental fixing is first.

The level of any fixing in the item name should be recorded.

Food added substances can be recorded either by their name or number.

Sustenance data board

Bundled food varieties have a sustenance data board that shows how much there is of:

Energy/kilojoules
Protein
All out fat
Immersed fat
All out sugar
Sugars
Sodium
Dietary fiber

These sums are given per serving, and per 100g or 100mL.

Tiny bundles, for example, spices, flavors, tea and espresso don't must have this board.

At the point when you analyze food sources, it's ideal to utilize the 'per 100g' segment.

Food organizations can pick their favored serving size, and that may be very not quite the same as what you would eat.

'Sugars' in the sustenance data board incorporate added sugars, as well as normally happening sugar.

It is critical that your kid gets the supplements expected for their turn of events. To set up a solid *eating regimen for your kid, you ought to think about the nourishing data of a food. In the event that you are uncertain about which supplements are essential for your kid, you can counsel the Australian Dietary Rules. You can likewise see your PCP.*

*Food added substances
Any added substances utilized in a food should be recorded in the fixings by*

their group name, for example,

Variety
Flavor
Humectant
Additive
Thickener
On the off chance that food varieties contain any hereditarily adjusted fixings, they will be marked with the words 'hereditarily changed'. This ought to show up in the item name

or close by the significant thing on the fixings list. All hereditarily changed (GM) food sources sold in Australia should go through a wellbeing test by Food Guidelines Australia New Zealand.

Wellbeing claims
A few food sources guarantee to have a particular medical advantage. This must be made for food varieties that

meet explicit nourishing rules.

The food should have a sufficient specific supplement either normally or added.

Cow's milk has sufficient normal calcium to guarantee it is a wellspring of calcium. Nonetheless, oat or soy drinks should add calcium to make wellbeing claims.

The food code forestalls organizations adding nutrients to food sources with poor dietary benefit.

Allergens
Food marks should contain data about normal allergens. These include:

Eggs
Fish and shellfish
Gluten
Milk

Peanuts

Sesame seeds

Soy

Tree nuts

Wheat and lupin

The fixings list should feature these food varieties. Moreover, sensitivity data ought to be proclaimed in a particular area on food marks, in strong text style.

Certain individuals with asthma respond seriously to sulphite additives. They should be recorded in the event that they are available in the food at a level that could cause concern.

it is essential to peruse food marks and check the fixings list while purchasing food

CHAPTER 7: QUICK AND EASY MEALS FOR PREGNANT WOMEN

Broiled vegetables with pesto crusted chicken or fish: Add a pesto-covered natural chicken bosom or fish filet (natural salmon or cod functions admirably) to a baking plate of part-cooked vegetables (for example new potatoes, cherry tomatoes, courgettes, onions, garlic red and yellow peppers) and cook for a further 10-20 minutes. Season with salt and newly ground pepper.

Chickpea and apricot tagine: To an essential pureed tomatoes (for example a tin of hacked tomatoes added to an onion and garlic clove mellowed in olive oil), mix in a portion of a finely cleaved red chill, a spot of ground cumin, a small bunch of slashed dried apricots and three modest bunches of slashed blended vegetables (for example carrots, courgettes and child corn). Add water on the off chance that important to make a pleasant sauce consistency, season and stew for 15 minutes. Add a tin of chickpeas and cook for a *further 10 minutes, then, at that point, mix in a modest bunch of new cleaved coriander and present with couscous, quinoa or earthy colored rice.*

Haddock poached in a parsley and lemon tofu sauce: Mix a portion of a block of luxurious tofu with a clove of garlic, the juice of around 50% of a lemon, some hacked parsley, salt and pepper. Add to a container with two haddock filets and gradually stew so the fish poaches (around 15 minutes, yet continue to check). Present with steamed broccoli or green vegetables and earthy colored rice.

Heated potato and yam filling thoughts:

Hummus (home-made preferably); Ratatouille or heated beans finished off *with ground Cheddar; Curds with chives or spring onion, blended in with cleaved red or yellow peppers, cucumber or prawns; Simmered vegetables and pesto; Tinned or smoked salmon blended in with curds or crème fraîche; Cannelini or margarine beans pounded with anchovy filets and dark olives, with lemon squeeze and dark pepper; Steamed leeks, broccoli or cauliflower florets blended in with cheddar sauce; Hard bubbled egg hacked and blended in with curds or crème fraîche and slashed parsley; Guacamole (once more, make your own or purchase in the store segment of your store)*

Flavorful Servings of mixed greens (ideal for a quick bite or pressed lunch):

A straightforward plate of mixed greens of blended leaves and cleaved crude vegetables can turn into a nutritious and heavenly dinner in minutes in the event that you keep your refrigerator supplied with shop enjoyments, for example, artichoke hearts, sun become flushed tomatoes, olives, hard bubbled eggs, peppers, sweet child peppers, anchovies, smoked fish and cuts of lean white meat. Smoked natural trout filet (a delightful option in contrast to smoked salmon that is loaded with Omega 3 Fundamental Fats) with flageolet beans or daintily steamed expansive beans blended in with lemon squeeze and dark pepper. Hot smoked natural trout or salmon, or smoked natural mackerel, chipped through entire grains, for example, *quinoa, earthy colored rice, millet or couscous, with cleaved crude vegetables. Season with lemon juice, balsamic vinegar, dark pepper and cleaved new spices.*

Tofu lumps (marinated in tamari or soy, ginger, garlic and sesame oil and earthy colored rice syrup), pan-seared for seven minutes or till brilliant and genuinely fresh. Throw through entire grains as above, or mix into buckwheat noodles with finely cut cucumber and ocean growth (parcels of dried assortments can be tracked down in the Oriental segment of grocery stores). Sprinkle with sesame seeds and serve warm or chilled. - Blended bean salad in with peppers, cherry tomatoes, red onion, sweet child peppers and hacked hard bubbled egg, with a tomato and basil dressing.

Chickpeas dressed with paprika, lemon juice, dark pepper and a sprinkle of ocean salt or Solo low sodium salt and parsley, with quinoa.

Warm potato salad with passata (sieved, hacked tomatoes - purchase at your general store), with a dressing produced using olive oil, paprika, chillies and squashed garlic.

Tabbouleh of couscous, bulgar wheat, millet or

quinoa with slashed cherry tomatoes, spring onions, cucumber, parsley, mint, olive oil, lemon squeeze and preparing.

Entire radishes, disintegrated feta cheddar, expansive beans and hay sprouts.

Blueberries and apricots on green leaves like sheep's leaf or spinach, with feta cheddar disintegrated over the top.

Simple PUDDINGS
Raspberry sorbet: Liquidize frozen raspberries and bananas to a smooth puree.
Apricot whisk: Puree a modest bunch of apricots (new or dried) with a portion of a cup of low-fat curd cheddar or smooth tofu eased up with two whisked egg whites.

CHAPTER 8: RECIPES FOR A HEALTHY PREGNANCY DIET

During pregnancy, your child eats what you eat - and depends on you to pick various good food varieties with fundamental supplements and nutrients. It's likewise vital to eat solid pregnancy dinners to keep your weight gain on target and lessen the gamble of pregnancy inconveniences. Furthermore, obviously, you believe that your dinners should taste astonishing! These flavorful and sound pregnancy recipes are loaded with supplements and have fiber, protein, and great fats to keep you feeling fulfilled.

Tortillas with yam, corn, avocado, cheddar, beans and lime

Between dealing with a solid weight gain, managing insane desires, and attempting to stay aware of your typical occupied plan, eating great during pregnancy can be a test. Be that as it may, stacking up on nutritious food is quite possibly of the smartest course of action for yourself as well as your child.

Get roused with these scrumptious recipes, which are sufficiently simple to handle on a weeknight and will fulfill your most impressive pregnancy hunger. These dinners are loaded with protein, supplements, and different advantages for yourself as well as your child.

Two glasses of water on the table, kale and dried organic product salad on a plate

Pregnancy recipes: Kale salad

There are a lot of motivations to cherish dim, mixed greens. Here is a major one, particularly from the get-go in your pregnancy: Kale is a great wellspring of folate. This B nutrient - known as folic corrosive in supplement structure - forestalls birth imperfections of the mind and spine in the principal trimester and supports your child's development all through pregnancy.

Past folate, kale is a superfood with nutrients and supplements that tackle normal pregnancy hardships, including fiber (to fight off craving and stoppage) and iron (to assist with forestalling frailty). This solid pregnancy dinner consolidates almonds for crunch and heart-sound unsaturated fat in addition to chewy dried figs for cell reinforcements and normal pleasantness.

Kale salad with dried organic product and toasted almonds

Dish loaded up with chard, red onion, bacon and feta

Pregnancy recipes: Frittata with chard

Protein is a significant cell building block, supporting your child's development all through pregnancy. Get a sound portion from eggs, which offer around 12 grams of protein for every serving of this frittata (about a fifth of your day to day prerequisite). One more in addition to: Eggs are one of the most mind-blowing dietary wellsprings of choline, which is significant for early mental health.

A sprinkle of milk and feta cheddar supply calcium to this pregnancy recipe, which fortifies your and your child's bones and teeth. Swiss chard adds a touch more calcium, in addition to

L-ascorbic acid to help your resistant framework.

Frittata with chard, red onion and feta

A plate and pot of ratatouille and prepared eggs

Pregnancy recipes: Ratatouille with eggs

Get the medical advantages of eggs (protein, choline, and that's just the beginning) in this solid pregnancy feast. It additionally has eggplant and tomatoes - both phenomenal wellsprings of potassium, which assists with keeping up with solid pulse. As a matter of fact, research recommends that remembering more potassium-rich leafy foods for your eating routine is a significant piece of a generally sound living technique to lessen the gamble of toxemia (hypertension during pregnancy).

Furthermore, tomatoes are a decent wellspring of L-ascorbic acid, which supports your resistant framework as well as assists your body with bettering retain iron from plant food sources like salad greens. That is particularly significant during pregnancy, since *your body needs iron to deliver blood to supply your child.*

Ratatouille with heated eggs

Broiled salmon, dried seeds and vegetables on a plate

Pregnancy recipes: Container burned salmon

Specialists at the Food and Medication Organization

(FDA) and the American School of Obstetricians and Gynecologists (ACOG) prescribe eating a few servings (around 8 to 12 ounces) seven days of low-mercury fish during pregnancy. Greasy fish like salmon is a top pick, since it's a brilliant wellspring of omega-3 unsaturated fats to help your child's mental health.

Protein-rich lentils make this dish super nutritious. This powerful little vegetable presents fiber (to keep you standard), folate (to safeguard against birth abandons), potassium (to help sound circulatory strain) and iron (to assist with forestalling iron-inadequacy weakness).

Container singed salmon with lentils and leeks

Combination of steamed vegetables on a plate

Pregnancy recipes: Steamed cod

Maximized on salmon and fish? Cod and other white fish can assist you with arriving at the a few servings of low-mercury fish suggested each week during pregnancy. While cod isn't as loaded with mind helping omega 3 unsaturated fats as different sorts of fish, it brags 17 grams lean protein in a 3-ounce, 71-calorie serving.

Various veggies make this pregnancy recipe a wholesome force to be reckoned with. Asparagus is a great wellspring of folate - straight up there with spinach - to assist with forestalling birth deformities of the mind and sensory system. Furthermore, artichokes are loaded with potassium for sound circulatory strain and fiber to assist with battling clogging.

Steamed cod with spring veggies

Barbecued chicken bosoms with spinach on a wooden plate

Pregnancy recipes: Barbecued chicken with pesto

Chicken very well could be your pregnancy protein of decision - for good explanation. Served skinless, chicken bosom is loaded with low-fat protein, at around 32 grams in a 3.5 ounce serving. It's additionally one of the most amazing creature wellsprings of potassium, to keep up with solid circulatory strain, and iron, to help the additional oxygen-rich red platelets you produce during pregnancy.

To flavor things up, this pregnancy pesto recipe utilizes pumpkin seeds instead of the standard pine nuts or pecans. Pumpkin seeds are one of the most strong normal wellsprings of magnesium, which assists *with glucose control and nerve working. Assuming pregnancy is meddling with your rest, there is even some proof that magnesium might help by directing synapses that control rest.*

Barbecued chicken with pumpkin-seed pesto

Combination of quinoa, barbecued shrimps and vegetables on a plate

Pregnancy recipes: Quinoa with shrimp

Shrimp are on the FDA's rundown of best low-mercury fish to hit your a few suggested servings each week during pregnancy. In a 3-ounce serving, shrimp offers 24 grams of protein in addition to a lot of circulatory strain advancing potassium.

Served on top of quinoa, this pregnancy recipe offers an additional portion of protein - a structure block of all of your child's cells. As a matter of fact, quinoa is one of few plant wellsprings of complete protein (meaning it contains every one of the nine amino acids the body expects to construct cells). An entire grain that is in fact a seed, quinoa is one more great wellspring of (possibly) rest advancing magnesium as well as folate to assist with forestalling brain tube deserts in your child.

Quinoa with shrimp, tomato and avocado

Three pots with chicken soup, farro and vegetables

Pregnancy recipes: Chicken soup with farro

Chicken soup is an evident solace food, and the farro in this solid pregnancy recipe gives it a charmingly nutty flavor. A customary Italian grain, farro coordinates impeccably with Italian-style cannellini beans, which are another supplement stuffed wellspring of protein, fiber, and iron.

Shitake mushrooms make this pregnancy recipe additional really great for you (and they make that appetizing, rich umami flavor). Those that are treated with UV lights are a wellspring of vitamin D (it will typically be noted on the bundle) to help safe and bone wellbeing.

Mushrooms are likewise a prebiotic, meaning they feed the solid microscopic organisms in your stomach to support your generally microbiome (the numerous *fundamental microorganisms that influence your wellbeing and, surprisingly, your mind-set).*

Chicken soup with farro and shiitake mushrooms

Two plates with barbecued pork tenderloin, blended vegetables and two glasses of water

Pregnancy recipes: Barbecued pork tenderloin

Other than being a fantastic wellspring of protein (at 22 grams in a 3-ounce serving) pork is a remarkable wellspring of zinc. This fundamental mineral backings a child's development and improvement during pregnancy as well as your invulnerable framework, which is more vulnerable to specific contaminations now that you're pregnant.

And keeping in mind that you're presumably generally acquainted with the medical advantages of entire grains like earthy colored rice or entire wheat, grain is comparatively an extraordinary wellspring of fiber, to keep your stomach related framework moving, and magnesium, to advance better rest possibly. This solid pregnancy feast consolidates chickpeas for one more portion of fiber, as well as folate (for sound mental health) and plant protein (to construct your child's cells). Dried apricots and currants add a blaze of sweet flavor in addition to supplements and sickness battling cell reinforcements.

Barbecued pork tenderloin with grain and dried apricots

Tacos with dark bean, yam, avocado and lime

Pregnancy recipes: Dark bean and yam tacos

Beans, the supernatural organic product - and a phenomenal vegan wellspring of child building supplements including folate, potassium, zinc, and iron. Their blend of fiber and protein additionally cooperate to assist with fighting off pregnancy desires.

This pregnancy recipe gets additional sustenance cred for the option of yams, which give you supportable, fiber-rich energy to upgrade the fulfillment factor. Like other orange products of the soil, yams are an *amazing wellspring of L-ascorbic acid, which assists you with retaining the plant-based iron in beans while assisting with building your child's bones and muscles and backing your resistant framework. Avocadoes are another superfood that presents significantly more folate and fiber in addition to tasty unsaturated fat.*

Dark bean and yam tacos with avocado

Bowl of chicken, curry and blended vegetables on the table

Pregnancy recipes: Yellow curry with chicken

Hoping to enliven supper time? Curry, a zest mix with turmeric, bean stew peppers, and that's just the beginning, is stacked with cell reinforcements and medical advantages for yourself as well as your child. Research proposes that these flavors might bring down glucose, which is helpful at any phase of life - yet particularly when you're pregnant.

Furthermore, on the off chance that you partake in the kind of curry, eating a greater amount of it currently: Doing so may assist with empowering a courageous eater later is great. Concentrates on show that amniotic liquid is enhanced with the food varieties in a mother's eating regimen. Infants are acquainted with these flavors during pregnancy each time they work on gulping a significant piece of amniotic liquid. As they develop, they might be bound to acknowledge (and appreciate!) flavors they got comfortable with in the belly. Attempt this recipe for an aiding of supplement stuffed yams, peppers, spinach, and chicken.

Yellow curry with chicken, spinach and butternut squash

Tofu, broccoli, rice and almonds on a plate

Pregnancy recipes: Tofu and veggie pan sear

Having a sound veggie lover pregnancy with just the right amount of additional planning is conceivable. Veggie lovers and vegetarians need to zero in on specific pregnancy-fundamental supplements and nutrients that aren't generally found in plant-based food varieties, including protein, iron, and calcium - which are all tracked down in tofu and other soy food sources.

Regardless of whether you're not vegan, adding more plant-based feasts to your eating routine has medical advantages for yourself as well as your child. Some exploration recommends that children of mothers who ate loads of plants during pregnancy are bound to eat these good food sources themselves *numerous years after the fact. This recipe knocks up the wellbeing factor with broccoli, snap peas, and earthy colored rice.*

Tofu, broccoli and sugar snap pan sear

Table loaded up with tortillas, guacamole, and container with steak fajitas

Pregnancy recipes: Steak fajitas

Fajitas are delectable method for adding more iron-rich red meat and veggies to your eating regimen. This recipe integrates flank steak, a less fatty cut with less calories and soaked fat as well as more protein than other red meats. It's barbecued - a better cooking strategy that secures in a fantastic smoky flavor.

This pregnancy recipe incorporates various other nutritious food varieties. Ringer peppers are stacked with L-ascorbic acid, with assists with the retention of iron to diminish the gamble of weakness (which is more normal during pregnancy). Supplement stuffed avocados are an incredible wellspring of filling unsaturated fats, potassium, folate, magnesium, choline, and then some. Furthermore, entire grain tortillas give you energy with a portion of obstruction battling fiber.

Steak fajitas with peppers and onions

Zucchini pasta on a plate

Pregnancy recipes: Zucchini noodles

While it's alive and well to go after the entire grain noodles all through your pregnancy, integrating veggie-based pasta into your standard fulfills pasta desires and work in additional veggies. Notwithstanding entire wheat pasta, this recipe utilizes cut zucchini, a great wellspring of vitamin A (as beta carotene) to help your child's eye improvement.

A nut-based sauce gets extra focuses for being both flavorful and supplement stuffed. It utilizes tahini (a sauce produced using sesame seeds) and peanut butter, which both proposition a portion of filling monounsaturated fats and fiber alongside cell reinforcement rich vitamin E.

Zucchini noodles with sesame sauce

Plate with cooked cauliflower steaks and yogurt in a little bowl

Pregnancy recipes: Broiled cauliflower

It probably won't appear as though a solitary vegetable could make a fantastic fundamental dish, however cooked cauliflower merits thought instead of the standard steak or chicken.

You might be shocked to find that its chewy surface thinks about to meat, and it's magnificent at engrossing different flavors. This pregnancy recipe matches it with a fiery Greek yogurt sauce for delightful Mediterranean flare.

Far better, cauliflower is a wholesome victor. It's an incredible wellspring of L-ascorbic acid, to support your safe framework and assist your body with retaining iron to diminish the gamble of weakness. It's likewise loaded with choline, which upholds your child's mental health, alongside folate, which forestalls birth imperfections of the cerebrum and spinal line.

Broiled cauliflower steaks with herbed yogurt

Solid breakfast on the table, avocado on toast, bubbled eggs, watermelon, cereal with blueberries and yogurt, carrots

CONCLUSION

The pregnancy diet cookbook is the ideal aide for moms to-be who need to furnish their children with the most ideal beginning throughout everyday life. From the nutritious recipes for every trimester to the thorough counsel on nourishment and way of life, this book has everything. Besides the fact that it gives delectable, sound recipes that are customized for each phase of pregnancy, yet it likewise gives significant data about nourishment, food handling, exercise, and way of life to help a positive pregnancy experience. Whether you are a first-time mother or a mother of many, this book will give you the information and recipes to guarantee a sound pregnancy and a blissful child. So get your duplicate of the pregnancy diet cookbook and begin your excursion on the way to a sound pregnancy today!